Simplified Solution Approach
To **ROSACEA**

Embrace Your Skin's Potential: Discover
Proven Strategies for a Vibrant, Even-Toned
Complexion and Renewed Self-Esteem

Dr QUENTIN GLYN

Table Of Contents

CHAPTER ONE

Rosacea

Rosacea is a long-term skin disorder that mostly affects the face. It is characterized by redness, visible blood vessels, and tiny red pimples that are filled with pus.

It often begins as a propensity to flush or blush more quickly than other individuals, and it may eventually lead to a persistent redness in the middle of the face that may eventually spread to the nose, cheeks, forehead, and chin. Although the precise etiology of rosacea remains incompletely known, it may arise from genetic predispositions, environmental triggers, or anomalies in blood vessels.

Because rosacea is a chronic condition with varying symptoms from person to person, managing it may be difficult. To properly control their symptoms, patients frequently undergo a variety of therapies, from topical drugs to lifestyle changes. Simplified solutions for rosacea aim to simplify this complex environment by offering simple, doable methods that people may include in their everyday routines.

An Overview Of Rosacea:

Recognizing rosacea's many symptoms and causes is essential to understanding the condition. Visible blood vessels, swelling red pimples, and redness on the face are typical signs. Individual differences may exist in triggers, which might include hot drinks, particular meals, sunlight exposure, alcohol, and stress. In extreme situations, rhinophyma—a thickening of the skin around the nose—can result from rosacea.

The unpredictability of rosacea may have a serious negative effect on a person's quality of life. In addition to its physical manifestations, the illness may also have psychological repercussions, leading to feelings of shame, self-consciousness, and in some cases, anxiety or despair. As a result, coming up with a simple remedy involves improving general well-being in addition to treating physical problems.

The Value Of An Approach To Simplified Solutions:

Patients may experience uncertainty and frustration due to the intricacy of managing rosacea. Simplifying solutions is essential to enabling people to manage their conditions well. People may discover particular triggers, take focused steps to relieve symptoms, and get a better understanding of their disease by condensing the abundance of information and treatment choices into a clear and understandable manner.

Additionally, a more straightforward method of treating rosacea promotes treatment consistency. Adherence to a simple strategy enhances the chance of lasting recovery, and chronic illnesses need continuing care. This method also recognizes that every person's experience with rosacea is unique and that there may not be a universally applicable remedy.

Objective And Range Of The Book:

This book's objective is to provide readers with a useful manual for controlling rosacea in their daily lives. The book seeks to demystify the disease, provide readers with information, and provide them with practical solutions for symptom management by providing a straightforward solution approach.

A thorough explanation of rosacea, including its origins, symptoms, and triggers, is covered in the book. It will examine the range of possible treatment alternatives, with a focus on those that can be readily integrated into everyday activities. We'll look at nutritional factors, skincare practices, and lifestyle adjustments so that readers may customize the strategy to fit their own set of circumstances.

The ultimate objective is to empower rosacea sufferers to take charge of their illness and enhance their quality of life. This book aims to be an invaluable tool for anybody navigating the difficulties of living with rosacea by providing knowledge in an understandable, practical, and quick way.

CHAPTER TWO
Recognizing Rosacea

Rosacea is classified as a chronic skin disorder that causes redness, visible blood vessels, and sometimes lumps on the faces that resemble pimples.

It usually affects the forehead, nose, cheeks, and chin, as well as the middle area of the face. Although the precise origin of rosacea is yet unknown, a mix of vascular, environmental, and genetic factors are thought to be involved.

Four Kinds May Be Distinguished In General From Rosacea:

The symptoms of erythematotelangiectatic Rosacea (ETR) subtype include flushing, persistent redness, and visible blood vessels.

Papulopustular Rosacea (PPR): PPR patients have redness that lasts a long time along with pimples that resemble acne. It's common to refer to this subtype as "adult acne."

Phymatous Rosacea: This uncommon kind is characterized by skin thickening, which often results in a bulbous appearance. Rhinophyma is the most typical location for this condition.

Ocular Rosacea: This subtype affects the eyes and produces symptoms including redness, irritation, and dryness. Ocular rosacea may manifest on its own or in conjunction with other skin complaints.

Causes and Triggers: Although the precise etiology of rosacea is unknown, a number of variables are thought to be involved:

Genetics: The disorder may have a hereditary tendency, as shown by family history.

Immune system dysregulation: Immune system anomalies may be a factor in rosacea-related inflammation.

Vascular Abnormalities: Prolonged redness might result from blood vessels near the skin's surface dilatation.

Demodex mites: Although their exact function is still being studied, these tiny mites that reside on human skin may be a factor in inflammation.

Although they might differ from person to person, frequent triggers for flare-ups of rosacea include:

Extreme temperatures, wind, and sun exposure are examples of environmental factors.

Diet: Alcohol, hot drinks, and spicy meals.

Emotional components: worry and tension.

Products for Skincare: Certain skincare and makeup ingredients may cause allergic reactions.

Common Symptoms: Depending on the subtype, rosacea symptoms may vary, however, they often consist of:

Facial Redness: A chronic redness that often resembles a sunburn.

Flushing: Sudden, transient episodes of redness.

Little red streaks on the skin are visible blood vessels.

Pimple-like Bump: These may have fluid within them (pustules) or be filled with pus (papules).

Sensitivity and irritation of the skin may result in burning or stinging sensations.

Dryness and Swelling: Skin, particularly the area around the eyes, may become dry and swollen.

Effect On Quality Of Life: Rosacea may significantly impair a person's mental health and quality of life in addition to their outward look. Visible symptoms have the potential to cause social disengagement, humiliation, and self-consciousness. Stress and worry may arise from the chronic nature of the illness and the possibility of flare-ups.

Rosacea patients may also feel physically uncomfortable as a result of symptoms like stinging or burning in their skin. The condition known as ocular rosacea may worsen the effects by irritating the eyes and impairing eyesight.

A comprehensive strategy is needed to manage rosacea, taking into account both the psychological and physical effects it has on people. To enhance general well-being, this may include medical procedures, lifestyle changes, and psychological assistance.

CHAPTER THREE
Subtypes Of Rosacea Identification

Determining the rosacea subtypes is essential to creating a focused and efficient treatment strategy.

Rosacea is a long-term skin disorder marked by redness in the face, visible blood vessels, and sometimes outbreaks that resemble acne. The subtypes aid in categorizing the particular symptoms an individual may encounter, enabling a more individualized method of treating the illness. The four primary rosacea subtypes are:

1. Rosacea Erythematotelangiectatica:

Signs:

Erythema, a persistent redness on the face that looks like a sunburn.

Telangiectasia is the term for visible blood vessels on the face, especially around the cheekbones and nose.

Hot feeling on the skin and flushing.

Recognition:

The visual appearance of prominent blood vessels and prolonged face redness is often used to make the diagnosis.

A dermatoscope may be used by medical practitioners to look more carefully at blood vessels.

Simplified Method:

Steer clear of things like alcohol, hot drinks, and spicy meals that might cause flushing.

Make use of a mild skincare regimen and stay away from harsh items that might irritate your skin.

Sunscreen is essential; use a broad-spectrum sunscreen every day.

2. Rosacea Papulopustularis:
Signs:

persistent redness accompanied by acne-like papules, which are tiny red pimples, and pustules, which are lumps filled with pus.

feelings of burning and flushing on the skin.

Recognition:

Lesions on the central face that resemble acne are necessary for the diagnosis.

Simplified Method:

Antibiotics may be used orally or topically to treat inflammation.

Use a gentle skincare regimen to prevent inflammation.

recognizing and avoiding situations that exacerbate symptoms.

3. Rosacea Phymatous:

Signs:

Thickening of the skin, which often results in a rough surface?

One of the most prevalent symptoms is enlargement of the nose (rhinophyma).

Recognition:

A diagnosis is often made based on the skin's obvious thickness, particularly around the nose.

Simplified Method:

For rhinophyma, surgical or laser techniques may be taken into consideration.

drugs to control the symptoms and stop them from becoming worse.

4. Rosacea Of The Eyes:

Signs:

Dry, red, and irritated eyes.

The feeling of something alien lodged in the eye.

swollen eyelids and, in extreme situations, even visual issues.

Recognition:

usually determined by an ophthalmologist using the patient's eye symptoms.

Simplified Method:

Synthetic tears to relieve parchedness.

To control inflammation, use oral antibiotics or antibiotic eye drops.

Maintaining clean eyelids might lessen symptoms.

For a precise diagnosis and individualized treatment plan, people with rosacea must speak with a healthcare provider. Although these streamlined methods provide broad recommendations, the intensity of symptoms and individual differences can need customized therapies from a medical professional. Furthermore, continuing care and lifestyle modifications are essential for the long-term treatment of rosacea.

CHAPTER FOUR

Environmental And Lifestyle Factors

Rosacea is a long-term skin disorder that mostly affects the face. It may cause redness, visible blood vessels, and, in some situations, little red pimples that resemble acne.

Although there isn't a treatment for rosacea, symptoms may be successfully managed by following a basic strategy that takes lifestyle and environmental variables into account. Here's a detailed explanation of the idea:

1. Nutrition And Diet:

• Trigger meals: There is evidence that certain meals and drinks may set off an exacerbation of rosacea. These might include meals rich in histamines, alcohol, hot drinks, and spicy foods. It's critical for people with rosacea to recognize and restrict their unique trigger foods.

• Anti-Inflammatory Diet: Prioritizing a diet high in fruits, vegetables, and omega-3 fatty acids that are anti-inflammatory may help lessen the inflammation brought on by rosacea. Foods that may be helpful include leafy greens, salmon, and flaxseeds.

• Hydration: Maintaining enough hydration is essential for healthy skin overall. Drinking enough water will help keep the skin hydrated and may even aid with symptoms.

2. Skincare Routines:

• Gentle Cleaning: Abrasive scrubs and harsh cleansers might exacerbate rosacea symptoms. Use a gentle cleanser without any smell and refrain from washing your face with hot water.

• Moisturization: It's critical to maintain moistened skin to avoid dryness, which exacerbates symptoms. To keep skin hydrated, use a hypoallergenic, non-comedogenic moisturizer.

• Sun Protection: Being in the sun may often aggravate rosacea. Sunscreen with a high SPF that is broad-spectrum can shield the skin from damaging UV radiation on a regular basis. It's also a good idea to seek shade and wear caps during the hottest parts of the day.

3. Environmental Stressors:

• Weather and Temperature: Severe heat waves or cold snaps may aggravate rosacea symptoms. It's important to shield your face in the winter and to stay out of the sun when it's hot outside.

• Wind and Humidity: Sensitive skin may get irritated by windy and humid weather. When the weather is bad, it might be beneficial to remain indoors and use face masks or scarves for protection.

4. Handling Stress:

• Mind-Body Techniques: Rosacea is often brought on by stress. Practicing stress-relieving techniques like yoga, meditation, and deep breathing exercises may help control symptoms.

• Enough Sleep: Sleep deprivation has an effect on skin health in general. Keeping a regular sleep schedule and making sure you get enough sleep are crucial for treating rosacea.

In summary:

For rosacea to be effectively managed, a streamlined solution approach that takes lifestyle and environmental aspects into account is important. People who have rosacea must emphasize stress management, recognize and avoid environmental irritants, pay attention to what they eat, and use moderate skincare techniques. Seeking advice from a dermatologist might provide tailored suggestions and interventions to improve the handling of rosacea symptoms.

CHAPTER FIVE

Comprehensive Methods For Rosacea Treatment

Rosacea is a chronic skin disorder that often has to be managed in a multimodal way. When it comes to treating rosacea, holistic methods—which take into account the individual as a whole rather than only concentrating on symptoms—have grown in favor. This strategy aims to treat the underlying reasons and enhance general health by including several facets of lifestyle, diet, and mental health. We'll discuss integrative medicine, natural remedies, mind-body practices, aromatherapy, and herbal solutions here as the four main pillars of holistic rosacea care.

Integrative medicine is the practice of combining complementary and alternative treatments with traditional Western medicine. This strategy entails working with medical specialists to develop a thorough treatment plan when it comes to rosacea. To treat the mental and physical components of the illness, dermatologists, dietitians, and holistic healers may collaborate. Prescription drugs, dietary adjustments, and lifestyle alterations are all possible components of integrative medicine.

Natural Medicines: A key component of holistic rosacea care is the use of natural medicines. Some people find that changing their diet and using certain supplements helps them feel better. For instance, including foods high in antioxidants, including berries, leafy greens, and fatty fish, may help reduce inflammation brought on by rosacea. Probiotics, zinc, and omega-3 fatty acid supplements could also be helpful. It's imperative that you speak with a healthcare provider before introducing supplements or making big dietary changes.

Mind-Body Techniques: Since stress is known to cause flare-ups of rosacea, mind-body techniques are crucial to comprehensive therapy. Deep breathing exercises, yoga, and meditation are a few practices that may ease tension and encourage calm. In order to enhance mental well-being and maybe lessen the frequency and severity of rosacea symptoms, mindfulness practices are very beneficial. Including these routines in everyday life may help reduce stress in general and improve rosacea treatment.

Herbal Remedies And Aromatherapy: Aromatherapy uses essential oils to support both mental and physical health. Certain essential oils, including lavender and chamomile, are well-known for their relaxing and anti-inflammatory qualities. Essential oils may irritate delicate skin, so it's important to proceed with care while using them. People with rosacea may benefit from herbal remedies having anti-inflammatory qualities, such as licorice root and green tea. Finding secure and efficient herbal medicines might be aided by speaking with a dermatologist or herbalist.

In summary, managing rosacea holistically entails taking a multifaceted approach to the problem. Whereas natural remedies concentrate on dietary and nutritional interventions, integrative medicine blends conventional treatments with complementary therapies. Stress is a frequent cause of rosacea, therefore mind-body techniques try to lessen it. Herbal remedies and aromatherapy are more choices for managing symptoms. Before making any big modifications to your treatment plan, always get advice from medical specialists.

CHAPTER SIX

Treatments For Dermatology

Rosacea is a long-term skin disorder that mostly affects the face. It may result in redness, visible blood vessels, and sometimes, the formation of tiny red lumps. Although there isn't a cure for rosacea, there are a number of dermatological treatments that may assist in properly controlling its symptoms. This is a comprehensive summary of rosacea dermatological treatments:

Topical Drugs:

Topical Antibiotics:

Goal: To manage microorganisms and lessen irritation on the skin.

Metronidazole, clindamycin, and azelaic acid are often used.

Application: Apply to impacted areas once or twice a day.

Topical Retinoids:

Goal: Encourage cell turnover to lessen inflammation and stop flare-ups.

Adapalene and retinolin are often used.

Application: As instructed by a dermatologist, usually administered in the evening.

Topical steroids for brief usage:

Goal: To promptly lower inflammation when flare-ups occur.

usage caution as prolonged usage may exacerbate symptoms and result in rosacea triggered by steroids.

Oral Drugs:

Antibiotics used orally:

Goal: Lower inflammation and manage bacteria in the body as a whole.

Doxycycline and Minocycline are Frequently Used.

Duration: Several weeks to months are usually the recommended duration.

Oral Treatments for Acne:

Use: For the treatment of papulopustular rosacea.

Isotretinoin is often used (in severe situations).

Be cautious: Because of possible adverse effects, close observation is necessary.

Short-term use of oral steroids:

Goal: A brief course of treatment may be used to address severe flare-ups.

usage caution: Due to negative effects, prolonged usage is not advised.

Light and Laser Therapies:

IPL, or intense pulsed light,

Goal: Addresses redness and visible blood vessels.

Procedure: Several sessions, spread out often by a few weeks.

PDL, or pulsed dye laser:

Goal: Reduces redness by focusing on blood vessels.

Procedure: Given in brief meetings.

Therapy using photodynamics (PDT):

Goal: Combine a photosensitizing agent with a light therapy.

Procedure: Targeting inflammatory blood vessels, the substance is applied to the skin and activated by light.

Expert Protocols:

Microdermabrasion:

The goal is to remove the outermost layer of skin, which improves texture and lessens redness.

Exercise caution: Only have a qualified expert do this.

Chemical Peels:

Goal: The skin is exfoliated to encourage regeneration.

Be cautious: For rosacea, superficial peels are usually advised.

Cryoprotection:

Goal: Freezes aberrant blood vessels and eliminates them.

Method: Applied with the use of a specialist tool.

Resurfacing using Lasers:

Goal: Lessens redness and enhances the texture of the skin.

Use caution: Needs experience to prevent symptoms from becoming worse.

It's important to remember that each individual may respond differently to therapies. A dermatologist's guidance and a customized strategy are necessary for the effective treatment of rosacea. A thorough rosacea treatment strategy should also include lifestyle modifications, recognizing and avoiding triggers, and adhering to a mild skincare regimen. For advice on the best course of action based on your unique requirements and symptoms, always see a healthcare provider.

CHAPTER SEVEN

Developing A Customized Skincare Program

For those who have rosacea, developing a customized skincare regimen is essential to controlling and reducing the condition's symptoms.

Rosacea is a long-term skin condition marked by flushing, redness, visible blood vessels, and sometimes pimples that resemble acne. A personalized skincare regimen may target certain issues and help calm and shield sensitive skin. Below is a detailed synopsis of every idea:

1. Moisturizing And Gently Cleaning:

Cleaning:

• Non-Irritating Cleansers: To prevent irritating skin, go for a gentle cleanser without any scent. Seek for formulas that are devoid of harsh chemicals and have a small ingredient list.

• Cleaning Method: Use lukewarm water to gently wash your face; avoid using hot water as this will make your redness worse. Rather than rubbing, use a gentle towel to pat the skin dry.

Hydrating

• Hypoallergenic Moisturizers: Choose moisturizers that are hypoallergenic and devoid of fragrances. Hyaluronic acid is one of the ingredients that may assist in moisturizing without irritating skin or clogging pores.

• Frequency: Always moisturize, particularly just after washing and before using any topical remedies. This aids in preserving the function of the skin barrier.

2. Sun Protection:

Sunblock:

• Broad-Spectrum Protection: Select a sunscreen that offers at least SPF 30 for broad-spectrum protection. People with rosacea often tolerate physical blockers like titanium dioxide or zinc oxide successfully.

• Reapplication: Reapply sunscreen every two hours, or more often if you perspire or have been in the water. Sunscreen is essential for avoiding flare-ups brought on by UV rays.

Extra Sun Protection Steps:

• Hats and Clothes: For further protection, think about wearing hats with broad brims and face-covering apparel.

• Steer Clear of Peak Sun Hours: The sun's rays are highest between 10 a.m. and 4 p.m., so try to avoid being in the sun during these times.

3. Selecting Products Suitable For Rosacea:

Products Free of Fragrances:

• Steer clear of Irritants: Select items that are marked as fragrance-free to steer clear of any irritants that can exacerbate rosacea symptoms.

• Formulas Without Alcohol: Avoid items with high alcohol content as they may cause irritation and drying out.

Ingredients that Reduce Inflammation:

• Soothing Agents: Seek for products with anti-inflammatory components such as green tea extract, aloe vera, or chamomile. These may lessen inflammation and redness.

Testing patches:

• Individual Sensitivities: Before adding new items to your regimen, do patch testing. This aids in identifying any possible sensitivities or triggers.

4. Tailoring A Schedule To Meet Specific Needs:

Recognizing Triggers

• Observational notebook: To find possible triggers, keep a skincare and lifestyle notebook. Spicy meals, alcohol, stress, and certain weather conditions are common causes.

• Cooperation with a Dermatologist: To identify and address specific triggers, carefully collaborate with a dermatologist. They may provide advice on certain substances or therapies that could be advantageous for your particular skin type.

Changing the Routine Based on the Symptoms:

• Flexibility in Routine: Be ready to modify your skincare regimen in response to your skin's condition at any given time. For example, you may want to streamline your regimen and concentrate on soft, calming items during flare-ups.

Expert Medical Care:

• Consultation with Dermatologist: Under the supervision of a dermatologist, investigate medical therapies such as laser therapy, antibiotics, or topical drugs. You may include them in your skincare regimen for more focused and efficient rosacea control.

Developing a customized skincare regimen for rosacea entails knowing your own triggers, choosing items that work for you, and modifying the regimen as your skin changes. Maintaining excellent contact with a dermatologist is essential to getting the best outcomes and controlling rosacea.

CHAPTER EIGHT
Handling Emotional Difficulties

In addition to treating the physical symptoms, controlling rosacea entails addressing the mental difficulties that come with having a chronic skin disease. Overcoming emotional obstacles is a crucial component of a holistic approach to rosacea management. This is a thorough examination of the ideas you raised:

Handling The Emotional Effect:

Recognizing the Emotional Effect:

Rosacea is a persistent, visible disorder that may cause emotional difficulties including sadness, self-consciousness, and humiliation.

Recognize and give meaning to your feelings. It's normal to experience emotional distress or frustration due to the way rosacea affects your look.

Learn for Yourself:

Understanding rosacea may give you confidence. A better understanding of the symptoms, causes, and available treatments may help reduce ambiguity and worry.

Interaction:

Be honest about your situation with friends, family, and coworkers. Inform them about rosacea to encourage sympathy and comprehension.

Putting Together A Support Network:

Looking for Expert Assistance:

See a dermatologist or other medical expert for advice on how to treat your rosacea. Their knowledge may provide light on available treatments and lifestyle modifications.

Getting Along with Others:

Connect with individuals who have experienced similar things by joining support groups, whether they are in-person or virtual. It may be reassuring and educational to share tales and counsel.

Including Close Relatives:

Help those close to you become knowledgeable about rosacea so they can provide understanding and support. Creating a solid support network at home is essential.

Strategies For Mental Health:

Techniques for Relaxation and Mindfulness:

To reduce stress, try yoga, deep breathing, or mindfulness meditation. These methods may support preserving emotional equilibrium since stress is often the cause of rosacea flare-ups.

CBT, or cognitive-behavioral therapy:

Developing coping mechanisms and correcting negative thinking patterns may be accomplished with the help of CBT. It facilitates a more positive emotional reaction and helps reframe ideas.

Creating Reasonable Objectives:

Divide more complex activities into smaller, more achievable objectives. Reaching little goals will help you feel more confident and adopt a more optimistic outlook.

Taking Care Of Oneself:

Skincare regimen:

Create a mild skincare regimen based on the requirements of your skin. Employ gentle, fragrance-free products and stay away from strong chemicals that might make your rosacea worse.

Choosing a Healthier Lifestyle:

Eat a healthy, balanced diet, drink enough water, and keep away from triggers like alcohol and spicy foods. These changes in lifestyle might improve your general health and complexion.

Treat Yourself:

Include in your routine the things that make you happy and relaxed. Self-care practices, such as reading, having a warm bath, or going outside, improve mental health.

Honor accomplishments:

No matter how tiny, recognize and appreciate your accomplishments. Recognizing the accomplishment of overcoming mental and physical obstacles is worthy.

In conclusion, managing emotional difficulties associated with rosacea requires a comprehensive strategy that includes self-care, mental health techniques, knowledge, and support. People may improve their entire quality of life and well-being by treating the physical and emotional elements of rosacea. Recall that creating a solid support network and getting expert advice are essential steps on your path.

CHAPTER NINE
Actual Success Stories

For those who suffer from rosacea, a chronic skin disease marked by visible blood vessels, redness on the face, and sometimes little red bumps, real-life success stories may be immensely motivating. Although there is no known treatment for rosacea, many individuals have used a variety of techniques to effectively manage their symptoms and have better skin. Here, we'll examine some recurring elements in these success stories, emphasizing effective tactics and the motivational tales of people who have seen a reduction in their rosacea symptoms.

Techniques That Satisfied Them:

Recognizing Triggers

Numerous testimonials highlight how crucial it is to recognize and stay away from factors that worsen rosacea symptoms. Alcohol, hot drinks, spicy food, and stress are common causes.

Since triggers might differ greatly from person to person, personalized trigger identification is essential.

Moderate Skincare Regimen:

Developing a mild skincare regimen is essential for controlling rosacea. Using gentle, fragrance-free cleansers and moisturizers is part of this.

Success stories often emphasize how important it is to use skincare products made especially for delicate skin rather than harsh ones.

Prescription Drugs:

Prescription drugs provided by dermatologists provide help for some people. These might be oral antibiotics, topical therapies, or other anti-inflammatory drugs.

Success tales often highlight how well medical treatments work to manage rosacea symptoms.

Changes in Lifestyle:

Incorporating stress-relieving activities like yoga or meditation into one's lifestyle may be quite helpful in treating rosacea.

Success stories often touch on the topic of sun protection, with people stressing how crucial it is to use sunscreen every day in order to avoid flare-ups.

Nutritional Modifications:

Success stories abound that talk about how food adjustments affect rosacea symptoms. Some people claim to feel better after cutting out certain items from their diet, including spicy or high-histamine meals.

Nutritional supplements—like omega-3 fatty acids—are often recommended as helpful dietary additives.

Motivating Trips For Clearer Skin:

Tenacity and endurance:

Numerous success stories emphasize how important it is to manage rosacea with patience and perseverance. Consistent work overtime is generally necessary to get clearer skin.

People talk about how they encountered obstacles but persisted in trying out various tactics until they discovered one that worked for them.

Education for Empowerment:

Success stories often include people learning about rosacea on their own. Those who are aware of the illness, its causes, and the various treatments are better equipped to make educated choices about their skincare.

Assistance Networks:

Creating a network of support is essential for many people dealing with rosacea. This might be consulting dermatologists for advice, joining support groups to meet others going through similar struggles, or asking friends and relatives for help.

Taking Care of Oneself:

Inspirational journeys sometimes include a change in focus toward self-care. This might include making everyday tasks more conscious, getting adequate sleep, and making time for enjoyable and relaxing activities.

Honoring Advancement:

Success tales highlight the value of acknowledging and appreciating little accomplishments. A positive outlook on the path to cleaner skin is aided by appreciating improvement, whether it be a decrease in redness or fewer flare-ups.

In conclusion, real-life success stories of people with rosacea management provide insightful information on the tactics that have helped them and the motivational adventures they have had. From recognizing triggers and implementing mild skincare practices to accepting lifestyle adjustments and establishing a support system, these narratives provide encouragement and useful advice for those managing the difficulties associated with rosacea.

Conclusion

In summary, managing the intricacies of rosacea necessitates a thorough and straightforward approach to solving the problem. We have covered many important ideas in this conversation with the goal of empowering those who are dealing with this skin issue. In closing, let's review the important elements, stress the value of taking charge, and provide support for a successful rosacea journey.

Summary Of The Main Ideas:
Recognizing and Steering Clear of Triggers: We have discussed the importance of

recognizing and avoiding triggers that aggravate rosacea symptoms. Through awareness of triggers like hot and cold meals, high-stress levels, and certain skincare products, people may successfully manage their disease in a proactive manner.

Gentle Skincare Routine: Using a gentle skincare regimen is essential for controlling rosacea. This entails selecting fragrance-free, gentle cosmetics and staying away from harsh chemicals that might irritate delicate skin. Sun protection, moisturizing, and gentle washing on a regular basis are essential for keeping skin healthy.

Holistic Lifestyle Changes: A balanced diet, frequent exercise, and stress management strategies are just a few examples of lifestyle changes that may greatly lessen the effects of rosacea. Adopting a holistic perspective on health may improve general well-being in addition to symptom relief.

Medical Intervention: Getting competent medical guidance is just as vital as making lifestyle improvements. Dermatologists are able to create customized treatment regimens that may include topical lotions, prescription drugs, or laser treatments. A coordinated effort between patients and medical experts guarantees a comprehensive and successful therapeutic plan.

Giving Readers The Tools To Take Charge:

At the heart of treating rosacea is empowerment. People need to understand that they can make good changes to their situation.

The reader may take charge of their rosacea journey by putting the knowledge obtained from knowing triggers into practice, establishing an appropriate skincare regimen, changing their lifestyle, and seeing a specialist.

As part of taking charge, proactive skin monitoring, keeping up with the latest advancements in rosacea therapy, and faithfully adhering to suggested skincare and treatment routines are also essential. This proactive approach encourages a feeling of agency over one's health and gives people the ability to actively engage in their own well-being.

Motivation For An Optimistic Rosacea Experience:

It might be difficult to start a new journey, but it's important to have an optimistic outlook. Appreciate the little things in life, like finding a trigger and avoiding it or seeing a change in the texture of your skin. Recognize that there may be setbacks in the progressive management of rosacea. Resilience and optimism, however, may greatly affect the whole experience.

Whether in-person or online, interacting with support groups may provide a feeling of community and common experiences. It may be encouraging and comforting to know that others have overcome comparable difficulties. Accept the trip as a chance for personal development, self-care, and self-discovery.

In conclusion, rosacea is a disease that may be properly handled with a comprehensive and straightforward treatment strategy, even if it may bring obstacles. People may start their road towards better, happier skin by grasping important ideas, taking charge of their health, and cultivating an optimistic outlook.

THE END